COMPLETE GUIDE TO UNDERSTANDING VARICOSE VEIN SURGERY

Expert Techniques, Recovery Tips, Prevention Strategies, Effective Treatment And Management For Optimal Relief

KLEIN HOYLE

Disclaimer

The content in this book is based on the author's expertise and comprehension of the topic. The author has no affiliation or link with any corporation, business, or person. This book is meant to give general information and educational material only, and it should not be interpreted as professional medical advice. Always seek the advice of a skilled healthcare expert if you have any queries about medical issues or treatments. The author and publisher expressly disclaim any responsibility resulting directly or indirectly from the use or use of the information included in this book.

Table of Contents

ABOUT THIS BOOK

The "Complete Guide to Understanding Varicose Vein Surgery" is an invaluable resource for anybody dealing with the complexity of varicose veins. This thorough book goes extensively into all aspects of varicose vein diseases and treatments, ensuring readers are well-versed in both non-surgical and surgical options. Beginning with a detailed introduction, This book explains what varicose veins are, delves into the many causes and risk factors, and emphasizes the symptoms and possible problems. It emphasizes the need for early diagnosis, laying the groundwork for comprehending the condition's course and consequences.

This book elaborates on the critical processes in detecting varicose veins, including physical tests and advanced imaging methods such as ultrasound and Doppler investigations. It also describes various diagnostic tests that are useful in obtaining an accurate and thorough picture of the vein's health, allowing for the development of an effective treatment strategy.

Nonsurgical therapies are extensively covered, including lifestyle adjustments, compression stockings, and sophisticated techniques such as sclerotherapy and laser therapy. Each strategy is thoroughly discussed, enabling readers to consider the advantages and disadvantages of each alternative. This section emphasizes the possibility of treating varicose veins without invasive surgery, providing hope to people seeking less aggressive therapies.

When surgical intervention becomes essential, This book provides a thorough explanation of the many alternatives accessible. This book covers everything from classic vein stripping and ambulatory phlebectomy to current procedures like endovenous laser therapy (EVLT) and radiofrequency ablation (RFA), ensuring that readers are up to date on the newest surgical advances.

Preparing for surgery is a key time, and the guide covers all of the important details, such as first consultations, pre-operative testing, and any required medication modifications. It also offers practical suggestions on how to prepare one's house for post-surgical rehabilitation, resulting in a smoother and more pleasant healing process.

On the day of surgery, This book provides clear instructions on what to anticipate, from pre-operative rituals to anesthetic choices and surgical process details. Immediate post-operative care is also discussed, allowing patients to control their expectations and reduce anxiety over the procedure.

Post-operative care is critical for a good recovery, and the guide covers everything from pain management to incision care, infection detection, and arranging follow-up visits. This section teaches patients how to make proactive efforts in their recovery path.

Recovery and rehabilitation are discussed, with a focus on activity limitations, exercise, physical therapy, and the timetable for returning to work and everyday life. This book also emphasizes the necessity of long-term treatment and preventative techniques for maintaining vein health and avoiding recurrence.

Potential problems and dangers connected with varicose vein surgery are openly acknowledged, with an emphasis on both frequent and uncommon but substantial hazards. The advice outlines ways to reduce these risks and gives clear guidance on when to seek medical assistance.

Finally, This book discusses long-term outcomes and maintenance, establishing reasonable expectations for results and offering advice on monitoring for recurrence. It promotes positive lifestyle modifications for vein health and emphasizes the significance of continued medical treatment and frequent check-ups.

Overall, the "Complete Guide to Understanding Varicose Vein Surgery" is a comprehensive and interesting resource that offers excellent insights and advice on all aspects of varicose vein management and treatment.

CHAPTER 1

Introduction To Varicose Veins

What Are Varicose Veins?

Varicose veins are swollen, twisted veins that may be seen just under the surface of the skin. They usually seem blue or dark purple and are most often seen in the legs. These veins form when the valves inside the veins, which normally assist control of blood flow back to the heart, become weakened or destroyed. As a consequence, blood collects in the veins, making them enlarged and twisted.

Varicose veins may form anywhere on the body, although they are more common in the lower extremities because of the increased pressure from standing and walking. They may cause discomfort, pain, and other serious health problems if not managed.

Causes And Risk Factors

Varicose veins originate from a mix of hereditary and environmental causes. Understanding this may assist in identifying high-risk people and adopting preventative interventions.

Genetic factors

A family history of varicose veins considerably enhances a person's chances of having them. Genetic predisposition influences the integrity of vein walls and the operation of vein valves, rendering certain persons more prone to the disorder.

Age

As individuals age, their veins lose flexibility and their valves deteriorate. This degeneration may develop in varicose veins, therefore age is an important risk factor.

Gender

Women are more prone than males to have varicose veins. Hormonal changes during pregnancy, premenstrual syndrome, and menopause might cause vein walls to loosen. Furthermore, hormonal medications, such as birth control pills, may heighten the risk.

Pregnancy

During pregnancy, the amount of blood in a woman's body grows while the flow of blood from the legs to the pelvis slows. This circulatory shift benefits the developing fetus but may also increase the veins in the legs. Hormonal changes during pregnancy also have an impact.

Obesity

Excess body weight puts strain on the veins, especially in the legs, which may lead to the development of varicose veins.

Prolonged Standing Or Sitting

Long durations of standing or sitting might reduce blood flow. Lack of activity may cause blood to pool in the veins, increasing the risk of developing varicose veins.

Lifestyle

A sedentary lifestyle and a lack of physical exercise may lead to impaired circulation, increasing the risk of varicose veins. In contrast, regular exercise may enhance leg strength, circulation, and vein function.

Symptoms & Complications

Recognizing varicose vein symptoms early may help you avoid problems and enhance your quality of life.

Common Symptoms:

• Visible veins are twisted and bulging, often blue or dark purple.

• Aching Legs: Pain or heaviness in legs after prolonged standing or sitting.

• Swelling occurs in the lower legs and ankles.

• Itching occurs around the damaged veins.

• Nighttime leg cramps.

Severe symptoms

• Skin Color Changes: Brownish discoloration around varicose veins.

• Venous ulcers around the ankles indicate serious vascular disease.

• Veins near the skin's surface may break and cause bleeding.

Complications

• Superficial Thrombophlebitis: Inflammation of the vein under the skin, producing discomfort and redness.

• Deep Vein Thrombosis (DVT) is a dangerous disorder where blood clots develop in deeper veins, increasing the risk of pulmonary embolism if they go to the lungs.

The Value of Early Diagnosis

Early detection of varicose veins is critical for avoiding complications and improving treatment success. Varicose veins are normally diagnosed by a physical examination and, in certain situations, ultrasound imaging to monitor blood flow and detect irregularities.

Benefits Of Early Diagnosis

• Early diagnosis and treatment of varicose veins may avoid serious consequences including venous ulcers and DVT.

• Early intervention may improve treatment outcomes and reduce invasiveness.

- Early symptom management improves quality of life by reducing pain, discomfort, and mobility concerns.

Diagnostic Methods

- During a physical examination, a healthcare professional checks the patient's legs for obvious evidence of varicose veins while standing.

- Ultrasound is an imaging technique that visualizes blood flow and detects valve function and vein clogs.

Individuals may successfully manage and treat varicose veins by first knowing what they are, recognizing the causes and risk factors, detecting symptoms, and highlighting the need for early detection.

CHAPTER 2

Diagnosing Varicose Veins

Physical Examination

A physical exam is the first step in detecting varicose veins. During this examination, a healthcare expert will visually evaluate your legs while you stand. The goal of this examination is to look for apparent symptoms of varicose veins, such as twisted, bulging veins in blue or deep purple. The examiner may also feel your legs for signs of pain, edema, or vein hardness.

The physical examination involves looking for symptoms of skin abnormalities associated with varicose veins, such as discoloration, ulceration, or dermatitis. Patients are often questioned about symptoms such as pain, heaviness, itching, or a burning feeling in the legs.

This information allows the practitioner to evaluate the severity of the ailment and its influence on the patient's everyday life.

In addition, the healthcare professional may do a manual compression test, which involves applying light pressure to the veins to see if blood flow is impeded. Observing how the veins react to pressure may help determine the level of venous insufficiency. This hands-on approach is required for an initial evaluation before progressing to more sophisticated diagnostic techniques.

Ultrasound Imaging

Ultrasonography imaging, particularly duplex ultrasonography, is an important diagnostic technique for assessing varicose veins. Duplex ultrasound combines standard and Doppler ultrasonography to provide visual pictures while also measuring blood flow in the veins.

This non-invasive examination gives a thorough picture of the anatomy and function of the veins in your legs.

During the operation, a gel is placed on the skin, and a portable equipment known as a transducer is moved over the desired region. The transducer generates sound waves that bounce off the veins, resulting in visuals on a display. These pictures aid in the detection of varicose veins, the direction of blood flow, and any reverse flow (reflux) that may be causing the veins to expand.

Duplex ultrasonography is very useful since it may identify the location of defective valves inside veins. Healthcare practitioners may establish a tailored treatment strategy by identifying areas where blood pools and fails to circulate effectively. This imaging approach is critical for mapping the venous system before surgical intervention or other therapies.

Doppler Studies

Doppler tests, a kind of duplex ultrasonography, are used to monitor blood flow inside veins. Doppler ultrasonography determines the speed and direction of blood flow by detecting variations in the frequency of sound waves reflected by moving blood cells. This information is critical for determining the efficiency of the venous system and detecting sites of venous insufficiency.

A Doppler study involves placing a transducer on the skin above the veins and transmitting sound waves. The instrument then records the reflected waves, which are translated into visual and audio information. The pictures and noises produced assist the healthcare professional in determining how effectively blood flows through the veins and if there are any blockages or reverse flow.

Doppler examinations may reveal aberrant blood flow patterns, such as reflux, which shows that the veins' valves are not working properly. This test is often combined with a physical examination and duplex ultrasonography to offer a thorough evaluation of the venous system. It is very effective for evaluating the degree of venous insufficiency and developing suitable treatment plans.

Other Diagnostic Tests

In addition to physical exams, ultrasound imaging, and Doppler investigations, various diagnostic techniques may be used to acquire a thorough picture of varicose veins. These tests may reveal more about the status of the veins and the underlying reasons for venous insufficiency.

Venography is a less frequent test that involves injecting a contrast dye into the veins and taking X-ray pictures. This examination may provide a thorough look at the venous system, revealing any blockages or anomalies. However, because of its invasive nature, venography is usually reserved for instances when other diagnostic approaches are inconclusive.

Another diagnostic method is photoplethysmography (PPG), which monitors changes in blood volume in the veins. This non-invasive test detects fluctuations in blood flow and venous pressure with light sensors put on the skin. PPG may assist assess the venous system's function and valve efficacy.

Air plethysmography is another approach for evaluating venous function. This test includes wrapping cuffs around the leg and monitoring changes in volume and pressure as blood flows through the veins. It gives useful information on venous capacity, outflow, and reflux, assisting in determining the level of venous insufficiency.

These additional tests, when paired with the core diagnostic procedures, provide a full examination of varicose veins.

Healthcare experts may effectively identify the illness and design an effective treatment plan suited to the patient's specific requirements by combining physical examination, imaging, and specialized testing.

CHAPTER 3

Nonsurgical Treatments

Lifestyle Changes

Lifestyle adjustments are essential for controlling varicose veins and may frequently greatly lessen discomfort. These adjustments are aimed at increasing blood circulation, lowering vein pressure, and keeping a healthy weight to keep the disease from deteriorating.

Exercise Regularly

Regular physical exercise is necessary for maintaining good blood flow in the legs. Walking, cycling, and swimming are very good. These workouts cause the calf muscles to contract, pushing blood back towards the heart and reducing vein pressure. Aim for 30 minutes of moderate activity most days of the week.

Maintain A Healthy Weight

Excess weight may put more strain on your veins, worsening varicose veins. Maintaining a healthy weight with a balanced diet and regular exercise might help relieve this stress. A diet high in fiber and low in sodium may help avoid edema and improve vascular health. Eat lots of fruits, veggies, healthy grains, and lean meats.

Elevate Your Legs

Elevating your legs many times during the day might assist relieve pressure in your leg veins. Try to raise your legs above your heart level for roughly 15 minutes many times each day. This is simply accomplished by lying down and resting your legs on pillows or a comfy surface.

Avoid Prolonged Sitting Or Standing

Long durations of sitting or standing may cause blood pooling in the veins. If your profession needs you to stand or sit for extended periods, take regular breaks to walk about and change postures. When sitting, avoid crossing your legs since it might reduce blood flow. For individuals who stand a lot, attempt to alternate your weight between one leg and the other regularly.

Wear Loose Clothes

Tight clothes, particularly around the waist, legs, and groin, might reduce blood flow. Choose loose, comfortable attire that doesn't confine your physique. This may enhance circulation and lower the likelihood of developing varicose veins.

Compression Stockings

Compression stockings are a key component of nonsurgical varicose vein therapy. They assist to increase blood flow, decrease edema, and alleviate symptoms like pain and discomfort. These stockings are available in a variety of compression levels, ranging from moderate to strong, and should be adjusted by a specialist to guarantee proper pressure and fit.

How Do Compression Stockings Work?

Compression stockings provide progressive pressure to the legs, tighter at the ankle and less constrictive at the top. This design promotes the upward flow of blood to the heart, decreasing blood pooling in the veins and lowering the risk of swelling and blood clots.

Types Of Compression Stockings

There are many forms of compression stockings, including knee-high, thigh-high, and full-length pantyhose. The decision is based on the location and severity of your varicose veins. In moderate circumstances, over-the-counter stockings may suffice.

However, in more severe situations, your doctor may recommend medical-grade compression stockings.

Using Compression Stockings

To get the most out of compression stockings, wear them appropriately. Put them on first thing in the morning, before getting out of bed, when your legs are the least swollen. Smooth out any creases or folds when putting them on, since these might cause pressure spots. Remove the stockings before going to bed, unless otherwise ordered by your healthcare practitioner.

Sclerotherapy

Sclerotherapy is a popular and efficient non-surgical option for small to medium-sized varicose and spider veins. It consists of injecting a solution directly into the afflicted vein, causing it to collapse and fade over time. This technique is minimally invasive and often conducted in a doctor's office.

The Sclerotherapy Procedure

Sclerotherapy is the injection of a sclerosant solution into a varicose vein using a tiny needle. The solution irritates the vein's lining, causing it to expand, cling together, and ultimately seal shut. The vein eventually goes away as scar tissue forms. The operation usually takes 15 to 45 minutes, depending on the number of veins treated.

Post-Operative Care

Following sclerotherapy, you will need to wear compression stockings or bandages to keep pressure on the treated veins and encourage recovery. Walking and being active may help prevent blood clots, but avoid hard activity for a few days. Some patients may have moderate soreness, bruising, or swelling, although these symptoms normally resolve within a few days to weeks.

Effectiveness And Results

Most patients see considerable improvement after a few weeks of therapy, however, many sessions may be necessary for the best outcomes. Sclerotherapy is very effective in eliminating varicose veins, although new veins might grow over time, necessitating further treatment.

Laser Therapy

Laser treatment is another non-surgical method for treating varicose veins, especially smaller veins and spider veins. This technique employs concentrated laser radiation to burn and destroy the afflicted veins, causing them to shut and fade.

Types Of Laser Therapy

There are two kinds of laser treatments for varicose veins: basic laser therapy and endovenous laser treatment (EVLT).

Simple Laser Treatment

Simple laser therapy is applied to the outside of the skin and is typically used for minor varicose and spider veins. The laser generates light energy, which is absorbed by the blood in the vein, causing it to heat and collapse. This technique is normally performed in a series of sessions, each lasting 15 to 30 minutes.

Endovenous Laser Therapy (EVLT)

EVLT is used to treat bigger varicose veins in the legs. During this treatment, a thin laser fiber is introduced into the afflicted vein via a tiny cut. The laser light burns the vein from the inside, forcing it to collapse and seal shut. The treatment typically lasts approximately an hour and is conducted under local anesthetic.

Post-Treatment Care And Outcomes

Patients may usually resume regular activities soon after laser treatment, however, excessive exertion should be avoided for a few days. Compression stockings may be prescribed to promote healing and enhance outcomes. Some individuals may endure minor bruising or pain, although these are typically transient. Laser treatment results are usually noticeable within a few weeks, however more sessions may be necessary for full vein elimination.

Individuals with varicose veins may successfully manage their disease and enhance their quality of life by learning about non-surgical treatment alternatives and making the appropriate lifestyle modifications.

CHAPTER 4

Surgical Options

Vein Stripping: Removing The Problem At Its Source

Vein stripping is a common surgical treatment used to treat varicose veins by physically removing the problematic veins from the body. It is normally done under general anesthesia, however, in certain circumstances, local anesthetic and sedation may be employed. This operation is often performed in a hospital or surgical facility.

During vein stripping, the surgeon makes tiny incisions around the groin and occasionally in the lower leg, depending on the size of the varicose veins. Through these incisions, a tiny, flexible wire is inserted into the afflicted vein.

Once the wire is in place, it is attached to the vein, which is then pulled out (stripped) of the leg.

Following vein removal, the incisions are closed with sutures or adhesive strips, and the leg is often placed in a compression bandage to promote healing and prevent swelling. The complete operation usually takes between one and two hours, depending on the quantity and severity of the varicose veins being treated.

Ambulatory Phlebectomy: Precision Removal Of Visible Veins

Ambulatory phlebectomy, also known as micro phlebectomy or stab avulsion, is a minimally invasive surgical procedure for the removal of superficial varicose veins at the skin's surface. Unlike vein stripping, ambulatory phlebectomy is conducted under local anesthetic and is commonly done as an outpatient procedure, so you may usually go home the same day.

The operation starts by designating the veins that will be removed. Then, small incisions, typically less than a quarter of an inch long, are made along the path of the targeted veins. Through these incisions, the surgeon inserts special hook-like equipment to grip and remove the varicose veins segment by segment.

One benefit of ambulatory phlebectomy is its accuracy. Scarring is minimized because the incisions are tiny and placed over the veins, leaving surrounding tissues completely unharmed. Compression stockings are often used after the surgery to promote recovery and minimize edema.

Endovenous Laser Treatment (EVLT): Using Light To Heal

Endovenous laser therapy (EVLT) is a minimally invasive method that seals varicose veins using laser light. This surgery is normally done as an outpatient with just local anesthetic.

During EVLT, a tiny laser fiber is introduced into the afflicted vein via a small incision near the knee. When the fiber is in place, it generates laser radiation that warms and seals the vein shut. This procedure leads the vein to collapse and then be absorbed by the body.

One of the primary benefits of EVLT is its efficacy and rapid recovery time. Many individuals may resume their usual activities after a day or two of the surgery. To get the best outcomes, follow post-procedure guidelines such as wearing compression stockings and avoiding extended sitting or standing.

Radiofrequency Ablation (RFA): Targeted Heat For Vein Closure

Another minimally invasive method for treating varicose veins is radiofrequency ablation (RFA), which involves sealing them up with heat produced by radiofrequency radiation. RFA, like EVLT, is often done as an outpatient procedure with just local anesthetic.

RFA involves inserting a tiny catheter into the afflicted vein via a small incision, generally around the knee. Once in position, the catheter sends radiofrequency radiation to the vein wall, causing it to heat up and collapse. Over time, the body absorbs the collapsed vein and redirects blood flow to healthy veins.

RFA has various advantages, including high success rates, low pain during and after the surgery, and a fast recovery period. Most patients may return to regular activities after a day or two, although intense exertion should be avoided for a short time.

Each surgical treatment for varicose veins has benefits and disadvantages. Vein stripping and ambulatory phlebectomy are more conventional surgical techniques, but endovenous laser therapy (EVLT) and radiofrequency ablation (RFA) are less intrusive treatments with shorter recovery periods and less pain. Discussing these alternatives with your doctor will help you choose the optimal treatment plan based on your specific requirements and preferences.

CHAPTER 5

Preparing For Surgery

Initial Consultation

The first step before having varicose vein surgery is to arrange an initial consultation with a vascular surgeon or vein disease expert. During this session, the surgeon will review your medical history, assess your symptoms, and do a physical examination of your legs. This evaluation may include ultrasonography to determine the degree of venous insufficiency and any underlying concerns.

The first meeting also allows you to ask questions and share your concerns with the surgeon. You may wish to learn about the many treatment choices available, the risks and advantages of surgery, and what to anticipate throughout the recovery period. It is important to be upfront and honest with your surgeon about your medical history, including previous operations, current medicines, and any allergies you may have.

In addition, the surgeon may discuss your surgical expectations and what results are achievable for your specific instance. This talk will assist ensure that you understand the process and the possible outcomes.

Pre-Operative Tests

Following the first meeting, your surgeon may conduct pre-operative tests to further assess your condition and confirm that you are fit to have surgery. These tests may include blood testing, imaging procedures like ultrasound or venography, and an electrocardiogram (ECG) to evaluate your heart function.

These tests are designed to discover any underlying health conditions that may need to be addressed before surgery and to assist the surgical team in planning the treatment appropriately. For example, if you have underlying heart disease or other medical issues, the surgical team may need to take additional care throughout the treatment to keep you safe.

In rare situations, further imaging examinations may be required to map out the veins in your legs and pinpoint the exact position of the varicose vein. This information will assist the surgeon in planning the surgical approach and selecting the most effective treatment procedure.

Medication Adjustments

Before surgery, your surgeon may prescribe medication changes to lower the chance of problems during and after the treatment. This might involve temporarily discontinuing some medicines that raise the risk of bleeding, such as blood thinners or nonsteroidal anti-inflammatory drugs.

If you have any chronic medical concerns, such as diabetes or hypertension, your surgeon may change your medicines to make sure they are under control before surgery. It is critical to closely follow your surgeon's instructions and tell them of any changes in your medication regimen.

Furthermore, if you are using herbal supplements or over-the-counter drugs, contact your surgeon since they may increase your risk of bleeding or interfere with anesthetic medications.

Prepare Your Residence For The Recovery Process

To provide a safe and pleasant rehabilitation environment following varicose vein surgery, you need to make certain changes to your living space. This might include:

1. **Arranging for Help:** Depending on the severity of your operation and your mobility, you may need help with everyday chores such as cooking, cleaning, and

bathing. Arrange for a friend or family member to assist you in the early stages of rehabilitation.

2. Creating a Restful Environment: Create a cozy recovery room with lots of cushions, blankets, and entertainment alternatives like books or movies. Elevate your legs as advised by your surgeon to relieve swelling and pain.

3. Stocking Up on materials: Make sure you have all of the materials you'll need throughout your recuperation, including bandages, dressings, pain relievers, and any assistive equipment advised by your surgeon, such as compression stockings.

4. Following Post-operative advice: Your surgeon will give you precise advice for caring for your wounds, controlling discomfort, and gradually returning to regular activities. Follow these steps carefully to enhance recovery and limit the chance of problems.

By following these measures to prepare for surgery and recuperation, you may help ensure that your varicose vein treatment goes smoothly and successfully.

CHAPTER 6

Day Of Surgery

What To Expect Before Surgery

Before having varicose vein surgery, it is important to prepare both psychologically and physically. Your surgeon will give you specific instructions on how to prepare for the operation, such as fasting for a particular amount of time before surgery, avoiding certain medicines, and arranging for someone to take you home afterward. To ensure a successful procedure, please follow these recommendations.

On the day of surgery, you'll usually check in at the hospital or surgical facility where the operation will be performed. You will be asked to change into a hospital gown and may be required to remove any jewelry or other accessories.

A nurse will check your medical history and vital signs to make sure you're ready for surgery.

Once you've settled in, your surgeon will most likely return to meet with you one more time to answer any last-minute concerns you may have and clarify the facts of the procedure. This is also an excellent opportunity to address any worries or reservations you may have regarding the surgery.

Anesthesia Alternatives

Varicose vein surgery may be conducted using several methods of anesthesia, depending on the technique and your personal preferences. The most frequent choices are local, regional, and general anesthesia.

Local anesthetic is the injection of a numbing drug directly into the region being treated, allowing you to stay awake yet painless during the process. This is often utilized for minimally invasive treatments like sclerotherapy or endovenous laser treatment.

Regional anesthesia numbs a wider region of the body, such as a complete limb, by combining local anesthetics with nerve blocks. This enables you to be aware during the treatment, but it may also be used with sedation to help you relax.

General anesthesia, on the other hand, induces a profound slumber in which you are entirely oblivious that the operation is taking place. This is usually reserved for more complicated treatments or for individuals who wish to remain asleep during surgery.

Your surgeon will review the various anesthetic alternatives with you ahead of time and assist you in selecting the one that best meets your requirements and preferences.

A Surgical Technique

The surgical method utilized to treat varicose veins will be determined by the location and severity of the veins, as well as your general health and medical history. Some of the most popular procedures are:

• Endovenous laser therapy (EVLT) is a minimally invasive method that includes introducing a tiny laser fiber into the afflicted vein and applying laser energy to heat and seal it shut.

• Sclerotherapy involves injecting a medicine directly into the varicose vein, causing it to collapse and fade away.

• \tVein stripping and ligation: In extreme situations, your surgeon may need to remove the vein via tiny incisions in the skin.

During the surgery, you will be comfortably positioned on the operating table, and the surgical team will take precautions to guarantee your safety and comfort throughout. Your surgeon will utilize specialized equipment and procedures to carry out the operation with accuracy and care.

Immediate Postoperative Care

After the procedure, you will be brought to a recovery area and carefully watched by nursing professionals. Depending on the kind of anesthetic used and the intricacy of the treatment, you may be required to remain in the recovery room for several hours or overnight.

During this period, the nursing team will monitor your vital signs, examine the surgery site for symptoms of bleeding or infection, and provide pain medicine as required. They'll also tell you how to care for the surgery site at home and when to see your surgeon for a post-operative checkup.

It is typical to feel some soreness and swelling in the days after varicose vein surgery, but this can generally be controlled with over-the-counter pain medication and compression stockings as prescribed by your surgeon.

Follow all post-operative instructions attentively to ensure a smooth recovery and the best possible outcomes.

CHAPTER 7

Post-Operative Care

Managing Pain And Discomfort

As your body recovers after varicose vein surgery, you may feel some pain and discomfort. Managing this soreness appropriately might help you heal faster. To assist relieve any discomfort you may be experiencing, your doctor will most likely prescribe pain medication. To achieve optimum efficacy while avoiding possible adverse effects, take these drugs exactly as prescribed.

In addition to medicine, there are various alternative ways to manage pain and discomfort. Elevating your legs might assist in relieving swelling and pain. Keep your legs up anytime you sit or lie down, preferably above the level of your heart. This improves circulation and relieves strain on your veins, which may relieve discomfort.

Ice packs or cold compresses may also assist in relieving pain and swelling at the surgery site. Wrap the ice pack in a towel to avoid direct contact with your skin, then apply it to the afflicted region for 15-20 minutes at a time, multiple times each day. This may help numb the region and decrease inflammation, bringing relief from pain.

It is important to listen to your body and rest as necessary. Strenuous activities and heavy lifting should be avoided during the first few weeks after recuperation since they might aggravate discomfort and slow healing. Instead, concentrate on soft motions and mild exercises to keep your blood circulating without overworking your body.

Care For Incisions And Wounds

Proper wound care is essential for avoiding infection and encouraging healing after varicose vein surgery. Your doctor will give you specific instructions on how to care for your incisions and wounds, but certain basic rules apply.

Keep the surgery site clean and dry to lessen the risk of infection. Avoid getting the incisions wet until your doctor gives you the okay to wash or bathe. When washing the area, use mild soap and warm water, then gently pat dry with a clean towel.

To avoid infection, your doctor may prescribe placing antibiotic ointment or a dressing on the incisions. Follow their directions closely and change the dressing as required to maintain the area clean and safe.

Incisions should be constantly monitored for symptoms of infection, such as increasing redness, swelling, warmth, or pus leakage. If you detect any of these symptoms, call your doctor right away, since early treatment is critical to avoiding problems.

You may suffer itching or pain as the incisions heal. Avoid scratching or picking at the scabs since it might impede the healing process and raise the risk of infection. Instead, use a moisturizing lotion or cream to soothe the skin and relieve irritation.

Identifying Signs Of Infection

Infection is a risk after any surgical operation, including varicose vein surgery. Recognizing infection symptoms early may assist in avoiding major problems and encourage speedier recovery.

Infection may be identified by increasing redness, swelling, warmth, or discomfort around the surgical site. You may also observe pus discharge or an unpleasant stench emanating from the site. In certain situations, you may have a fever, chills, weariness, or body pains.

If you observe any of these symptoms, call your doctor immediately. They may need to give antibiotics or other treatments to eliminate the illness and keep it from spreading.

In extreme situations, more medical intervention may be required to treat the infection and facilitate recovery.

In addition to keeping an eye on the surgery site for symptoms of infection, you should also consider your general health and well-being. Eat a balanced diet, remain hydrated, and get enough rest to help your body recover naturally. Avoid smoking and drinking since they might slow recovery and raise the risk of problems.

Follow-Up Appointments

Follow-up visits are an important element of the post-operative treatment for varicose vein surgery. These visits enable your doctor to check on your progress, evaluate your recovery, and address any concerns or difficulties that may emerge.

Your doctor will arrange your first follow-up visit soon after your surgery, usually within a week or two.

During this session, they will examine your wounds, remove any stitches or staples as needed, and review your healing progress. They may also use imaging tests, such as ultrasound, to assess the surgery's success and guarantee proper blood flow.

Follow-up sessions will be made as required, depending on your specific recovery and any lingering problems. It is important to attend all planned visits and discuss freely with your doctor about any symptoms or problems you are having.

Prepare to address any changes in your symptoms, new or worsening pain, or any questions you may have concerning your recovery at follow-up sessions. Your doctor is there to assist and guide you throughout the recovery process, so don't be afraid to ask questions or get clarification on any part of your treatment. By being involved and proactive in your post-operative care, you may assist in guaranteeing the greatest possible result and long-term success from your varicose vein surgery.

CHAPTER 8

Recovery And Rehabilitation

Activity Restrictions

After varicose vein surgery, it is essential to adhere to specified activity limits to promote optimal healing and reduce the risk of complications. Your doctor will give you comprehensive advice customized to your specific condition, but here are some general rules to remember.

First, avoid excessive activity or heavy lifting for the first two weeks after surgery. This includes activities like jogging, weightlifting, and strenuous aerobic workouts. These activities might put pressure on the surgical site, causing it to take longer to recover.

It's also important to avoid sitting or standing for lengthy periods, since this may put strain on the veins and slow circulation.

If your profession requires you to sit or stand for long periods, try to take regular breaks to move about and stretch your legs.

Additionally, avoid bathing in hot tubs or saunas, since heat may exacerbate swelling and pain. Choose lukewarm showers instead, and avoid exposing the surgery site to direct sunlight, which may increase the risk of scarring.

Finally, follow your doctor's suggestions for compression stockings or bandages. These garments improve circulation and minimize swelling, which aids in the healing process. Wear them exactly as advised, and do not remove them until your doctor expressly instructs you to.

Following these activity limits can assist in guaranteeing a smooth recovery and reduce the chance of problems after varicose vein surgery.

Exercise And Physical Therapy

While it is critical to relax and avoid heavy activity immediately after varicose vein surgery, adding light exercise and physical therapy into your recovery plan may enhance healing and improve long-term results.

Your doctor will offer specific instructions depending on your situation, but here are some broad suggestions to consider.

Begin with mild exercises, such as walking or light stretching, as soon as you feel comfortable. These exercises assist to improve circulation and avoid blood clots, which are typical consequences after surgery.

As you heal, progressively increase the intensity and length of your workouts. Swimming, cycling, and yoga are wonderful low-impact exercises that enhance circulation without placing too much pressure on the surgery site.

Some individuals may benefit from physical therapy, particularly those who have underlying muscular weakness or mobility difficulties. A physical therapist may design a tailored workout program to suit individual requirements while also restoring strength and flexibility.

However, you must listen to your body and avoid pushing yourself too hard, particularly in the early phases of recuperation. If you encounter pain or discomfort while exercising, stop and see your doctor.

Exercise and physical therapy may help you recover faster and enhance your overall health and well-being.

Returning To Work And Daily Activities

Returning to work and regular activities after varicose vein surgery marks a big milestone in your rehabilitation. However, it is critical to handle this shift with caution to guarantee a seamless and effective return.

Your doctor will make specific suggestions depending on your unique circumstances, but here are some broad ideas to keep in mind.

First, think about the physical demands of your employment and how they may affect your rehabilitation. If your work demands heavy lifting or lengthy periods of standing, you may need to take extra time off or temporarily change your tasks.

It's also important to listen to your body and take pauses when required. If you feel any pain or discomfort while doing your professional tasks, take a break and visit your doctor if required.

When returning to work, consider things like transportation and schedule. If feasible, organize transportation to and from work to reduce stress and avoid sitting or standing for extended amounts of time.

Consider making alterations to your desk to improve comfort and circulation. To alleviate leg strain and improve posture, consider utilizing a standing desk, ergonomic chair, or footrest.

Finally, be gentle with yourself while you adjust back to work. It is natural to feel weary or exhausted when you return to your usual schedule, so emphasize self-care and listen to your body's needs.

Following these suggestions and speaking honestly with your employer and healthcare team will guarantee a successful return to work and everyday activities after varicose vein surgery.

Long-Term Care And Prevention

While varicose vein surgery may significantly alleviate symptoms, it is critical to take precautions to avoid recurrence and preserve long-term vein health. Here are some recommendations for long-term care and prevention.

First and foremost, have a healthy lifestyle by eating a well-balanced diet, exercising frequently, and avoiding smoking. These practices improve overall vascular health and lower the likelihood of developing new varicose veins.

In addition, exercise excellent vein hygiene by elevating your legs while resting, avoiding crossing your legs when sitting, and using compression stockings if your doctor recommends them.

Regular follow-up visits with your doctor are also required to evaluate your vein health and treat any issues or symptoms that occur.

Finally, be aware of variables that may increase your chance of developing varicose veins, such as weight, pregnancy, and extended standing or sitting. Take precautions to reduce these risk factors, such as keeping a healthy weight, using compression stockings during pregnancy, and taking frequent breaks to walk about if you have a sedentary job.

Implementing these tactics into your everyday routine will help avoid recurrence and maintain good vein health after varicose vein surgery.

CHAPTER 9

Possible Complications And Risks

Common Complications

Varicose vein surgery, like many medical procedures, has certain hazards. Minor problems may include bruising, edema, or soreness at the surgical site. These symptoms usually disappear on their own with time and adequate treatment. However, in certain circumstances, more serious issues may develop.

A typical consequence is the development of blood clots, commonly known as deep vein thrombosis (DVT). This happens when blood clumps together inside a vein, usually due to restricted mobility after surgery. Symptoms of DVT include swelling, discomfort, and redness in the afflicted leg. If you encounter any of these symptoms, get medical assistance immediately to avoid severe consequences.

Another possible consequence is surgery site infection. While infections are uncommon, they may arise after varicose vein surgery, particularly if adequate cleanliness procedures are not followed. Infection symptoms may include increasing pain, redness, warmth, or discharge from the incision site. If you observe any of these symptoms, call your doctor right away for a correct diagnosis and treatment.

Additionally, some individuals may have nerve injury or numbness in the treated region. This might be due to surgical manipulation or irritation of surrounding nerves during the surgery. While nerve injury is usually transitory, you should notify your doctor if you have persistent numbness or weakness.

Rare But Severe Risks

Although uncommon, varicose vein surgery has more significant hazards. One such danger is severe bleeding, which may happen during or after the treatment.

While surgeons take steps to reduce bleeding, some circumstances, such as underlying medical problems or drug usage, might increase the risk. In extreme circumstances, heavy bleeding may need further intervention or blood transfusion.

Another uncommon but dangerous risk is injury to deeper veins or adjacent tissues during surgery. While contemporary procedures seek to reduce this danger, unintentional harm to neighboring arteries or nerves may still occur in certain situations. Such injuries may need further surgical intervention or specialist therapy to resolve.

Furthermore, allergic reactions to anesthesia or other drugs used during surgery are conceivable but rare. Allergic responses may vary from minor symptoms like itching or rash to more serious ones like trouble breathing or anaphylaxis. Patients who have a history of allergies or drug reactions should notify their doctor before surgery to reduce this risk.

How To Minimize Risk

While varicose vein surgery has certain hazards, you may take action to reduce them. To begin, verify that the surgery is performed by a trained and experienced surgeon. Check out their qualifications, experience, and patient reviews to ensure you're in skilled hands.

Follow all pre-operative instructions from your surgeon, including any food or drug restrictions. This may include abstaining from some drugs that raise the risk of bleeding, such as aspirin or blood thinners, in the days leading up to surgery.

During the surgery, talk freely with your surgical team and report any unexpected symptoms or concerns right away. After surgery, carefully follow the post-operative care recommendations, which include adequate wound care, activity limits, and the use of compression garments as advised.

Attend all planned follow-up sessions with your surgeon to track your recovery and treat any possible issues early on. By following these precautions and actively engaging in your treatment, you may help reduce the risks associated with varicose vein surgery.

When To Call Your Doctor

It is critical to recognize the signs and symptoms that may signal a problem after varicose vein surgery. If you encounter any of the following, call your doctor right away:

1. Excessive bleeding that does not stop under pressure.

2. Swelling, redness, or warmth in the affected limb may suggest a blood clot.

3. Persistent pain or discomfort that becomes worse with time.

4. Signs of infection include increasing redness, edema, or discharge from the incision site.

5. Numbness, tingling, or weakness in the treated region persists.

Prompt contact with your healthcare practitioner is critical for prompt diagnosis and treatment of any issues that may emerge. If you have any worries about your recovery or well-being after varicose vein surgery, get medical assistance right once.

CHAPTER 10

Long-Term Outcomes And Maintenance

Expected Results

Patients who have varicose vein surgery should expect to see a considerable improvement in their symptoms and looks. The major purpose of the procedure is to relieve pain, and edema, and improve the esthetic look of the afflicted veins.

Patients may endure soreness and bruises shortly after the operation. However, as the healing process advances, these symptoms usually subside. Patients should notice a decrease in discomfort, edema, and the appearance of bulging veins with time.

The long-term outcomes of varicose vein surgery are typically excellent. Many patients report a significant improvement in their quality of life, including a decrease in symptoms such as leg discomfort, heaviness, and weariness. Furthermore, the surgery's esthetic advantages, such as smoother, more beautiful legs, may improve self-esteem and general well-being.

Monitoring For Recurrence

While varicose vein surgery may give long-term treatment for many individuals, other people may experience recurrence. Patients must be careful in monitoring their symptoms and getting medical assistance as soon as they discover any indicators of recurrence.

Regular follow-up meetings with a healthcare practitioner are critical for determining the long-term success of the procedure. During these sessions, the doctor will analyze the patient's recovery, and any residual symptoms, and look for evidence of vein recurrence or complications.

Patients should also be proactive in maintaining excellent vein health by adhering to their doctor's advice for lifestyle adjustments and self-care techniques. Patients who are aware and sensitive to their bodies' cues may help avoid recurrence and retain the advantages of surgery in the long run.

Lifestyle Changes For Vein Health

In addition to varicose vein surgery, patients may benefit from implementing lifestyle modifications to improve vein health and lower the chance of recurrence. These lifestyle changes may complement surgical therapy and improve long-term results.

One important lifestyle modification is to maintain a healthy weight with a well-balanced diet and frequent exercise. Excess weight may increase pressure on the veins, aggravating varicose vein symptoms and raising the likelihood of recurrence. Patients who achieve and maintain a healthy weight might relieve pressure on their veins and enhance circulation.

Another crucial part of vein health is to remain moving and avoid sitting or standing for lengthy periods. Regular activity promotes good blood flow and prevents blood from collecting in the veins. Patients should try to integrate regular activity into their daily routine, such as walking, swimming, or cycling, to maintain their veins working properly.

Ongoing Medical Care And Check-Ups

Even after varicose vein surgery, patients must continue to get continuing medical treatment and monthly check-ups to ensure optimum vein health. These follow-up sessions enable healthcare practitioners to track the patient's progress, treat any concerns or difficulties, and provide advice on long-term care.

During check-ups, the doctor may do diagnostic procedures such as ultrasound imaging to examine the status of the veins and detect any symptoms of recurrence or problems.

Based on the results, changes to the patient's treatment plan may be suggested to guarantee sustained success.

Patients should also be upfront with their healthcare practitioner about any changes in their symptoms or general health. Patients who remain proactive and involved in their treatment may collaborate with their medical team to resolve any difficulties as soon as possible and maximize their long-term results after varicose vein surgery.

Conclusion

Finally, both patients and healthcare practitioners need to have a thorough grasp of varicose vein surgery. This complex operation, which aims to alleviate the pain and possible health hazards associated with varicose veins, requires careful consideration of many elements before, during, and after the surgery.

First and foremost, people considering varicose vein surgery should communicate openly with their healthcare practitioners. This conversation should include the underlying reasons for their varicose veins, accessible treatment choices, and the possible risks and advantages of surgery. Understanding these characteristics allows people to make more educated choices regarding their healthcare experience.

Furthermore, rigorous preoperative examinations are required to confirm each patient's appropriateness for surgery.

This usually includes a thorough medical history review, a physical examination, and diagnostic procedures like ultrasound imaging to determine the amount and severity of the varicose veins. Identifying any underlying illnesses or contraindications allows healthcare practitioners to adjust the surgical approach to each patient's specific requirements.

Varicose vein surgery uses precision procedures to treat underlying venous insufficiency while avoiding trauma and optimizing cosmetic results. The fundamental objective, whether using classic surgical treatments like vein ligation and stripping or minimally invasive techniques like endovenous laser ablation or radiofrequency ablation, is to eradicate dysfunctional veins while maintaining healthy venous circulation.

Postoperative care is critical to maintaining maximum healing and long-term success after varicose vein surgery. Patients are usually recommended to wear compression stockings, elevate their legs, and participate in regular physical exercise to improve blood flow and lower the risk of problems like deep vein thrombosis or recurrent varicose veins. Routine follow-up sessions enable healthcare practitioners to assess the patient's progress, address any concerns, and make any required changes to the treatment plan.

In addition to treating the physical symptoms of varicose veins, it is important to acknowledge the psychological influence that this illness may have on patients' quality of life. Varicose vein surgery not only alleviates physical problems but also boosts self-esteem and confidence, helping people to take control of their looks and well-being.

Finally, a thorough knowledge of varicose vein surgery requires a multifaceted approach that takes into account the medical, surgical, and psychological components of treatment. Healthcare practitioners may achieve optimum results and enhance the overall quality of life for patients with varicose veins by

providing them with information and support
throughout their treatment journey.

THE END

www.ingramcontent.com/pod-product-compliance
Lightning Source LLC
Chambersburg PA
CBHW051908250726

48659CB00002B/532